JOURNEY
TO
INFINITY

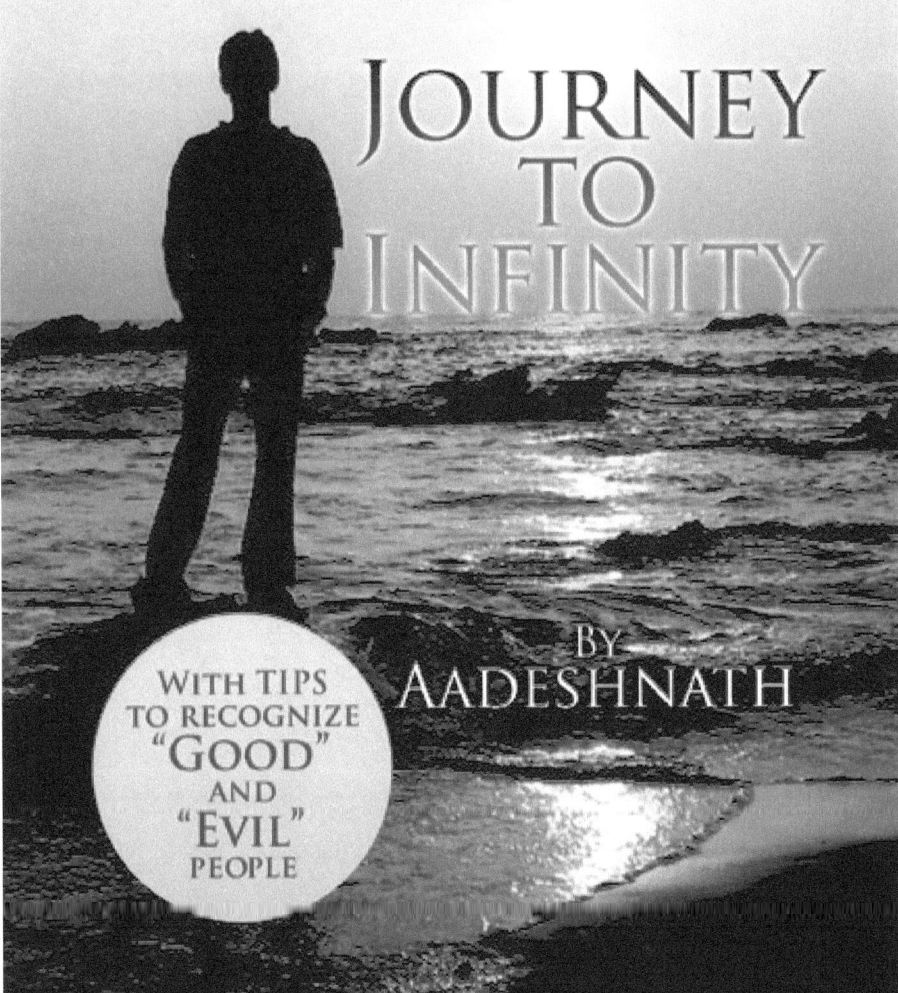

A HYBRID OF RELIGIOUS THOUGHT
FROM BHAGWAD GEETA, BIBLE AND QURAN THAT SPEAK
TO STRESSFUL LIFE IN NORTH AMERICA.
EXPERIENCE THE CALMNESS WITHIN!

JOURNEY TO INFINITY

BY AADESHNATH

WITH TIPS
TO RECOGNIZE
"GOOD"
AND
"EVIL"
PEOPLE

Author Contact
Yogi Hemant Panchpor alias Aadeshnath
37 Miller Street
Toronto-ON-M6N 2Z6
Tel: 001- (416) 653.8125
E-mail: hemantpanchpor@hotmail.com

To order additional copies of this book, contact:
Xlibris Corporation
1-888-795-4274
www.Xlibris.com
Orders@Xlibris.com
49197

|| Aum Nav Nathay Namo Namah ||

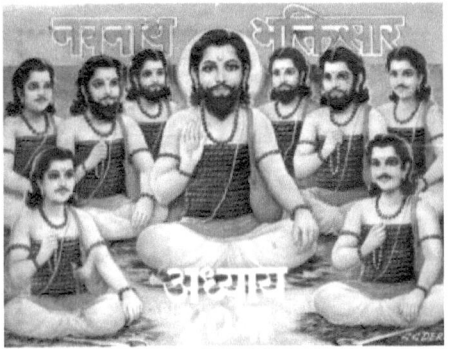

Nine Incarnations of Lord Vishnu,
Nav Nath, during 13th century

|| Aum Matrudevay Putrudevay cha Namo Namah ||

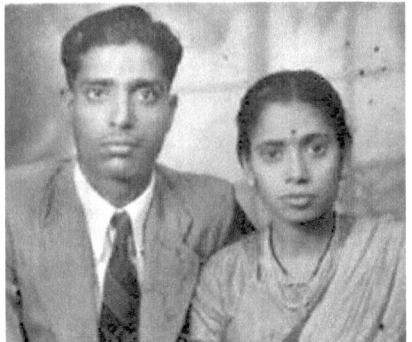

Father and mother, late Mr. Ramachandra
and Smt. Shalini Panchpor

|| Aum Gururdevay Gururpatnyai cha Namo Namah ||

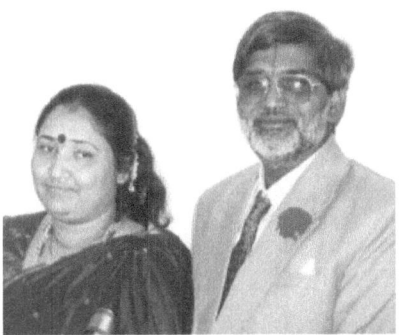

Mr. Ramdas alias Narendranath and Mrs. Rekha Kamble

Contents

FOREWORD

This book attempts to find solutions to problems in North America caused by stress in everyday life. The stressful conditions that individuals face are due to general conditions in the society. There is fundamental difference between the way of life in the East and the West. Though the conditions in the West seem to be favorable for personal development and successful materialistic life, peace of mind is missing in the fragmented society due primarily to existence of distrust.

This publication is dedicated to Ashley alias Teshwarie Persaud, a girl from Guyana who settled in Toronto. She is an example of a typical girl from North America. In this way, this book addresses the problems faced by the people in the North America who lose their faith in society and live a life without school education as a result of social conditions and stress due to lonely lives.

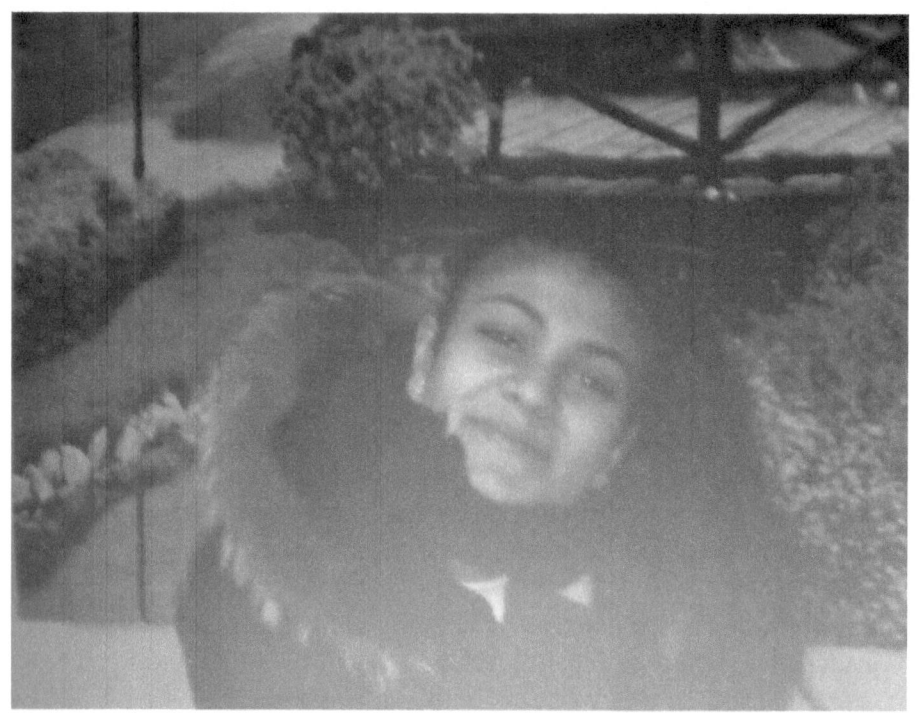

This book is a result of divine inspiration after seeing Ashley Persaud's struggle due to negative and positive spiritual energies.

Hope, intelligent people from the West, will welcome this publication!

Yogi Hemant Panchpor alias Aadeshnath
Author
2nd January, 2008

Author's Note

Today I went to Silverthorn Library on St. Clair Avenue West and asked a library assistant about books on Yoga. While I was talking to her, I was shocked to learn how much disinformation about Yoga exists in Toronto. When I read a few books written by the Western Yoga practitioners, I realized that Yoga has been considered as an option to Health Club exercise, which, in fact, is not the case. Yoga is an ancient science from India, and Holy Bhagwad Geeta itself is a part of Upanishada written on Brahmavidya (Knowledge of Universe) under the category of Yogashastra (Science of Yoga).

As one of my friends puts it, "Yoga in the West is just like having sex as against making love and taking care of the beloved person". I am sorry to quote the sentence in language used by him, but, unfortunately, the knowledge of Yoga from India has been taken out of its context and the culture in the West. Though the action involved in both the cases is the same, you get satisfaction and mental peace when you make love, but not when you have sex, though your organ may get temporary relief like that from drugs. The real happiness and mental peace come from making love and getting ready to lose something, if necessary, for that person. The sort of Yoga accepted in the West is like the former but to reap the benefits of achieving mental peace and happiness leading to Moksha (or liberation from rebirth cycles, as accepted by Hindus), it is necessary to look at it as the later. Mental Yoga that forms the foundation of yogic exercises is very important in understanding the concept of Yoga. Please note that Mental Yoga by Andy Bernstein or Dr. Mark Hyman is different.

People from the West go to India for a few months for training in Yoga, and then start teaching Yoga in their respective countries. It is a good service for people and a nice way of earning money. Yogis, who spend their life learning Yoga, could not master yogic practices to reach the end (i.e. Moksha). It is, therefore, unwise to say that learning Yoga at a Yoga Studio can give you all the same benefits. Nav Nath, one of the spiritual communities in India, aims to achieve Moksha with the help of Yoga and yogic practices. The former refers to postures and the later refers to other methods to achieve mental peace and happiness. Most of the literature published in the field of Yoga pertains to Yoga postures and not Mental Yoga that is the basis of learning Yoga. This is the first attempt of publishing a book on Mental Yoga with Nav Nath principles. There is a lot of knowledge hidden either in Sanskrit or in the local languages or possessed by the Gurus and Sadhakas of spiritual branches in India.

I am thankful to Ashley, Tanya, Nargis, Rani, Christina, Carolyn, Joy, Jay, Dev, Shivaram, Jagdish, Brij, Obaidullah, Javed, Shabir, Ashar, Azzra, Zakir, Josesh, Mark, Jim, Terry, Philip, Greg, Darryl and many others for inspiration, discussion and help in compilation of this book, though the book remains a divine inspiration!

I hope, intelligent people from the West, will welcome this publication!

Yogi Hemant Panchpor alias Aadeshnath
Author
2nd February, 2008

CHAPTER 1

Where the West Meets the East

What the East Thinks of the West

Typically, when we think of the East without the national boundaries but by the way of thinking process, there is a common link among the countries of the East. The East consists of many countries right from Japan, China almost up to Middle Eastern countries. The East does not include Australia, New Zealand and parts of Middle Eastern countries that do not have influence of the culture from the East. In the East, typically family ties are more important than material success. The people in these countries think that the West is more materialistic in approaches to the life. In fact, wherever the people from the East visit or migrate, they brought with them thinking patterns from the East. In order to live peacefully in the West, they have accepted the Western way of life, which is generally intellectual and practical in approach. The West has always welcomed the new thoughts in order to enrich life. Eastern people have transformed their material life to match the Western societies; however, social and spiritual inclinations of Eastern people have hardly changed.

What the West Thinks of the East

It is equally important to understand what the West thinks of the East. The West typically consists of many countries from America and Europe, and Australia, New Zealand as well as other countries that are not included in the East. African countries seem to have absorbed both Eastern and Western influences as they typically inherit the thought and social life of family ties from the East though their approach to the life is typically Western. Typically, the West thinks of the East as poor countries with large populations, low literacy rates and low standards of living except in economically advanced countries that have imitated Western life and have commercial relations with the West. Understanding the importance of huge emerging markets, especially India and China, the West has taken steps to explore the Eastern countries by way of economic co-operation and enlarging commercial and military influence. The troubles in Islamic countries like Afghanistan and Iraq have always attracted the West in an effort to know more about these societies. The conflict starts between the West and the East when the West tries to overpower the East.

Conflict Between the West and the East

The conflict between the West and the East is for freedom of thoughts and actions at social level. The East often expressed their feelings through different forums like United Nations. Behavior or action (Achar), thoughts (Vichar) and Speech (Ucchar) are interconnected. All actions are generally the results of mature thoughts after repeatedly spoken requests. The conflict can only be settled temporarily by means of military or economic power, however, difference of opinions and actions will create new conflicts and hatred will continue.

Religion and Conflict

Generally speaking, conflicts of interest have always been based on religious difference, though amazingly no particular religion allows attacking innocent people of other religions except in self-defense. The basic core principles of different religions are the same. However, interpretations by followers through religious practices are different. Human beings through Divine mandate have created religions with different approaches to life. Religion conversion is not a solution to this conflict. Solutions can be found in patterns of thinking that generally govern the individual religions. Now the question remains whether it is possible to transform religious thinking, so that there can be harmony rather than conflict in and between the West and the East.

Changing Religious Thinking

There have been efforts to change the way different religious practices look at the life in order to bring peace and harmony in society, especially in the East where many different religions co-exist. In the West, such efforts have been made for understanding comparative religion, and as such, have academic interest rather than social importance. Social change is brought through economic policies in the West. Now that core principles of all religions are same, the question arises why there are conflicts. Many religions have two basic forces of 'evil' and 'good'. Interestingly, every force thinks that the other is 'evil' and it is 'good'. When this game is over, conflict will end.

How to End the Conflict

The question is how to change thinking process when it is almost unanimously agreed that thinking is individualistic rather than group based. In both the West and the East, there are people who take advantage of difference in the way of thinking pattern for their personal interest and gain. In fact, religion plays an important role to make thinking a group activity. There are growing numbers of people, especially in the West, who do not attach themselves to a religion and live life based on economic needs. The difference in the thinking is generally attributed to the cultural background, which in turn, based on group thinking of the religious teachings and practices. Thus, religion remains only medium of hope for peace on earth, as there are majority of people who believe themselves as religious and follow religious way of living life.

What are the Differences in Religions

Now that we know there is similarity in the core principles of different religions, it is worthwhile to explore the differences that remain the basic cause of conflict. There are many religions, and parts of a religion that believe in certain way of life and practice religion differently. Differences in religions are attributed to differences in the customs followed by each religion. The major similarity in all religions is existence of 'good' and 'evil' forces.

What is Yoga

Yoga, in terms of postures, helps millions of people to live peaceful life even in the stressful conditions in the West. Unfortunately, since Yoga has been considered as an option to physical exercise, it has been combined with other options such as Therapeutic Yoga and Polaris Yoga. The very purpose of Science of Yoga (Yogashatra) has been lost in this fusion, resulting in much confusion. Peace and happiness being the outcomes of Yoga, have been replaced by fusion and confusion (Maya). In the East, many similar concepts have emerged over the period that emphasizes the importance of meditation and other metaphysical practices. Concept of Yoga became known from Hindu literature, namely Bhagwad Geeta. Patanjali, a great thinker and scholar from the East, has outlined some principles of Yoga called "Patanjali Sutra". Bhagwad Geeta defined Yoga as a state of mind (BhagwadGeeta-Ch.2-v-48). Patanjali further used body postures to harmonize body and mind actions. Though it looks at human life in four tiers viz. physical, mental or emotional, intellectual and spiritual, it tries to harmonize with next tier in increasing order from physical to spiritual. It continues the harmonization until all the four tiers are completely saturated with harmony and is called 'yogic' state of mind. It is believed in Hindu community that a human being is released from rebirth cycles and gets Moksha if he dies in this state.

Yoga from Bhagwad Geeta

The Bhagwad Geeta defines 'Yoga' as the knowledge leading to 'Viyog' or separation from sorrow or a state of happiness and bliss (Ch.6-v-23) and looks at Yoga as a state of mind that is not affected by external conditions consisting of success and failure, achievement of objectives and attachments to the results in terms of benefits and gains (Ch.2-v-48). Mind is governed by brain through intelligence, wisdom i.e. acquired intelligence through experience, ego and conscience. There is a wide belief based on Bhagwad Geeta, that one can achieve Moksha during the life rather than after death (Ch.5-v-27-28). 'Yogi' wins his own conscience and achieves balanced state of mind when the differences of emotions like coldness and hotness, happiness and sadness, honor and insult cease to exist. His brain is full of knowledge from both Atmagyan or Spiritual Science and Vinyan or Natural and Social Science, and earth soil, stone and gold are all equal to him (Ch.6-v-7-8). The doer's authority is limited to doing Karma but does not extend to results in terms of benefits and gains (Ch.2-v-47). Yoga increases concentration through meditation and, in turn, enhances favorable results. The peace and happiness can be achieved by detachment from worldly pleasures of satisfying senses and organs, which, in fact, are reasons for the sorrowful conditions in life (Ch.5-v-21-22). Western life is based on expectations and action-reaction process and focuses on satisfying worldly pleasures, and thus results in sorrowful conditions. According to Bhagwad Geeta, a person has two parts *viz.* 'Prakruti' or nature, which is the feminine part, and 'Purusha' or soul, which is the masculine part of human body. Prakruti has three manifestations in behavior:

- Satva, referred to as 'good' in many religions.
- Tamas, referred to as 'evil' in many religions.
- Rajas, reflects human expectations as a middle layer between Satva and Tamas.

The results are assured by natural process (Prakruti) of action and reaction, and not by God (Purusha). The ignorance among people overcomes this knowledge, and confusion prevails (Ch.5-v-14-15). The soul is different from Prakruti, and is referred to as Purusha or Atma, that is confined in the body and controlled by Prakruti(Ch.13-v-19-22).

Why Prakruti and Purusha are Important

Prakruti controls behaviour, and Purusha controls Prakruti in the similar manner as a man and a woman function in normal human life. Pratruti needs Purusha, and Purusha needs Prakruti as they are complementary as man and woman. Harmony in society is brought through co-existence of men and women to continue life through the reproduction process. Similarly, harmony in the body and mind is achieved through balance of Prakruti and Purusha. First three tiers of Yoga viz. human body, emotions and mind, intellect and wisdom represent Prakruti, and the fourth, soul represents Purusha that is responsible for spiritual needs.

How Human Body Qualities are Determined

There is wide belief in Hindu society based on Bhagwad Geeta (Ch.13-v-21) that during sexual intercourse between man and woman (Purusha and Prakruti), all the four tiers (i.e., body, mind, intellect and soul) are in harmony. Rajanisha or Osho from Pune, India thinks that through sexual activity also one can achieve Infinity or 'yogic' state of mind (i.e. Samathi or Moksha). Actually, during sexual intercourse, there is interplay of all the four tiers with spiritual energy, both negative (i.e. hatred, cruelty and destruction) and positive (i.e. love, compassion and construction), being transmitted from one person to other reflecting changes in the thoughts in a woman during reproduction process. In fact, there is a wide spread belief in Hindu society that the egg upholds the characteristics that are prevalent during sexual intercourse, and as such, good thoughts during sexual intercourse lead to a baby that carries these good thoughts. Positive spiritual energies are emitted at places of worship like temples, churches, mosques and gurudwaras. Negative people through their negative thoughts and actions spread negative spiritual energies.

Soul and Spirit

Atma or soul refers to powerful kinetic energy that drives intellect, wisdom, mind, body and senses through ego and conscience, thus it is superior to objects, organs, mind and wisdom (BhagwadGeeta-Ch.3-v-42). Dhruti or spirit refers to potential energy that drives mind, body and soul (BhagwadGeeta-Ch.18-v-33-35).

Conceptual Difference to Life

There is a conceptual difference in approaches to life between the West and the East. To the West, human is 'a wanting animal' as Management Guru puts it, and all the theories are based on expectations of human animal and managing the human being through controlling the expectations. No wonder then, the human behaves as an animal. To the East, however, a human being is 'a spiritual being', and physical expectations are necessary but not important. In the East the people are happy without fulfilling their basic needs. Some people are happy living on the donations given by society at the temple as they believe that God has provided them with food; and return the favor (cost of food) by providing selfless service to people in need or doing some job at temple without any monetary return. The people who offer free food are grateful to those who accept their share of donation as an opportunity to clean their sins. In the West, there are people who live on Food Bank, but they are not happy, as they believe that it is their inability to provide themselves with food and need to live on charity of other people. The Eastern approach to the life has been challenged by GATT and international trade after 1990s; however, there is fundamental mental difference in the Eastern outlook.

Why the West is Facing Trust Problems

The approach to life is the reason why Western society has been facing problems of distrust or ill faith. In the West, in almost every walk of life negotiations are carried out based on the false show of not wanting something even though there is a need and want for that activity or product. This works in many situations when the negotiations are used. However, though physical need can be satisfied with this approach, the trust that comes from the spiritual need is not built. While people can physically achieve many milestones in the life, they are spiritually deserted. Distrust is the apparent manifestation of this spiritual desertedness. In the West, money can get one what one wants, the same is not true for trust. Mutual trust is the result of spiritual alignment rather than physical togetherness though the later is necessary for the former. Trust is the basis of all human relationships, but there are many relationships in the West that lack mutual trust and respect. The East refers to such relationships as Maya or false hallucination. (BhagwadGeeta—Ch.7-v-25)(Quran—Ch.3-v-185-186)

Why Trust is the Basis of Life in the East

In the East, many relationships are based on trust rather than the money involved in the deal. It is evident from the fact that if someone helps somebody in the East, that person remembers the help and surely returns the favor. However, in the West, many people speak sweet and convincing language to get the help and forget the person once their need is fulfilled. In fact, after coming to the West, even Eastern people follow the similar way of life, and change themselves to the Western conditions. Thus, in the West, those who do well physically and mentally are generally not doing well materialistically; and those who do well materialistically have often physical or mental problems due to distrust. There are very few people who are doing well materialistically and also physically and mentally happy.

Dilemma of Life

In fact, imbalance between physical and mental happiness and materialistic success is the dilemma of life in both the West and the East. Western life is result-oriented, and means adopted to achieve result are not important. Though favorable results produce a successful materialistic life, peace and happiness are not gained. However, in the East, result is not important but the means adopted need to be fair. The 'fair means' provide peace and happiness, but not necessarily a successful materialistic life. Materialistic success, to some extent, is based on mental peace and happiness. For balancing this physical and mental happiness Yoga is useful. Yoga helps to balance body and mind through physical 'exercise' as well as mental 'innercise'. Physical exercise refers to physical postures of Yoga and other yogic practices that keep the body healthy and fit, and mental innercise refers to the changing mental framework for the approach to the life by way of Mental Yoga. Yoga of posture, as accepted in the West, is incomplete without Mental Yoga. The concept of Mental Yoga is based on selfless service or seva. In the West, results determine the success of the endeavor. Result oriented working fashion dictates the means, whether appropriate or not. Until the results are assured, people don't care about the means adopted. There is difference between unlawful activities and immoral activities. Unlawful activities are punished, not immoral activities. Until you are not caught, you are smart. Some people take advantage of the gaps in the laws and keep exploiting people and authority. These unscrupulous people make authorities helpless. In addition to a good legal system without holes, concept of Yoga is necessary for mental happiness and keeping mental balance in case of failure.

Problems in the West

The problems that are common in the West are lies, loss of good spiritual behavior, excessive importance assigned to money and materialistic needs and consequences thereof such as violence, distrust, lack of collective society and excessive importance to individualistic needs rather than social needs. Thus, the Government does not have direction for social changes but it directs itself by economic objectives. The people, in general, live in fear, which some believe to be the driving factor of life.

Problems in the East

The problems in the East are somewhat similar to the West as the East is following the Western way of life. Violence is common in both these places. However, the East has more spiritual awakening and trust in the society than in the West. There is a collective society in the East in the first place as a result of following religious thinking. That can also become a problem if there is friction among different parts of a religion or different religions. The poverty in some parts of the East is due to confusion in the minds of people. Some people believe that they cannot change their life by way of action and that their life events are pre-determined due to fate. Thus, for many people in the East, hard work is not important as in the West.

Solutions to Problems of the West and the East

The only solution to the problems of the West and the East is changing the thinking process. Though this change in thinking in the West and the East is different as their thinking patterns are different, the way the change can be brought in is also different. However, the medium to bring about that change is same and that is Yoga. Let's see when the West meets the East!

CHAPTER 2

When the West Meets the East

World Political Conditions

The present political conditions in the world are quite volatile, both in the West and the East. The West is engaged in military action in some parts of the East. Though Bush has started the 'war on terrorism', the concept is not new to some countries in the East.

World Economic Conditions

The West is facing recession or slow economic growth with either a cash crunch or a credit crunch. The East, on the other hand, has been engaged in rapid economic development and high economic growth. To some extent, the growth is due to cash inflows from the West. At the same time, there is sizable difference in the growth rate between the West and the East. In both the West and the East, there are high inflationary trends making the life of common people miserable.

Islamic Way of Life

The Islamic way of life today is going through a radical social change. The intellectuals in the Islamic world are not able to convince the fundamentalist faction in their society. The intellectuals cannot voice their opinions openly and in a free and democratic manner as they fear the fundamentalists will eliminate them either by assassination or by any other means of threats. Though the process of social change has been started, it is not yet finished. It may take a few generations to make that change happen.

Hindu Way of Life

Hindu society has started a social change process in eighteenth century when many scholars from India visited the Western countries, and changed the society after going back to India. Some, however, preferred to live in the West and are contributing to the economies of the West. At present, the Hindu society is also on a verge of change. Thus, the change is continuous and generally follows the Western way of life. Hindu society, for simplicity includes Sikhs, Jains, Buddhists and other Hindu people of Indian origin and other countries like Nepal and Sri Lanka.

Christian Way of Life

At present, Christians all over the world have realized the power of 'service to human being', either for the purpose of religious and economic considerations or to make an impression on the society. In the West, however, Christians are fractured in their collectivity due to excessive freedom of thoughts and individualistic ways of living. Though social change is evident, many people are not concerned about the society. Also, many Christians prefer to stay away from the religion and lead an independent life unlike Hindus and majority of Islamic people.

Process of Globalization

The process of globalization started in 1990s has great impact not only on the economic life of the people but also on the religious beliefs of the people all over the world. Though the process started to use the available resources of the world effectively and efficiently, the process has far greater impact on the cultures of different countries. For example, in a country like India, where in the past people believed in living a simple life with peaceful means and preserving culture of the country with no excessive accumulation of wealth has now changed. Globalization has changed the face of this country resulting in the richest man of the world coming from India. The change in the thinking process also affects culture and religion.

The 21st Century and the Possibility of a 3rd World War

The 21st century has brought in the concept of Internet when the computer has reached to the billions of poor people of the world. Thus, the competition for wealth accumulation using Internet has increased tremendously in the world. Obviously, there is a tussle among rich and poor countries of the world for power sharing. Generally, the process of power sharing leads to the world war. The economic conditions in the West are also indicative of rapid financial changes.

Time for the West and the East to Meet

The time at present is characterized by meeting of the West and the East. The process of understanding and negotiation is already started for preservation of culture of preference. This process has led to adoption of Yoga by the Westerners and the stressful life of the West by the East in order to live a comfortable materialistic life.

When the West Meets the East

The process of hybridization of West and the East has started. The author believes, based on his intuition, the result of the process will be seen some time in 2010 when the people of the world would be going through great change of thinking and struggle for power.

CHAPTER 3

How the West Meets the East

Process of Meeting

The process of meeting remains the same, whether it is meeting a partner, a friend or even a Guru or a teacher, as the process invariably involves the exchange of thoughts and ideas. The process of globalization has given a kick-start to the process of exchange and is not only limited to goods and services, but also thoughts and ideas. New businesses are getting set up at different parts of the world to make the transfer of these exchanges easier and smoother. Technology of the West has already reached the East; whereas the spiritual ideas and the human resources of the East are reaching to the West. This process enables the exchange of the best practices and methods around the world.

What the East has to Offer

For the West, the East has many facets of life to offer. The first and foremost is human resources for routine jobs in customer service using telephone lines or specialized jobs like Information Technology projects as it is economically beneficial to the West due to low salaries. Oil and gas have been traditionally imported from the Middle East. China has become the 'factory of the world' due to low cost of raw material, cheap skilled workers, technologically advanced machinery and detailed knowledge of requirements from the West. Spiritual Gurus come from the East in addition to the specialized techniques and knowledge in the disciplines of health care and other services useful in stress reduction. Yoga in the physical form (i.e. postures) is very popular in the West. Ayurveda for herbal medicine as well as Ashram for spiritual advancement are very well accepted by the West. Many practices like Reiki, massages and other Chinese techniques are also in great demand in the West.

What the West has to Offer

The West is providing economic base for the Eastern countries by way of foreign direct investments in businesses. Foreign multinational companies are entering the East due to the huge markets with high return on investments and high demand for products in those markets. Financial companies have already entered in the first phase. Now, the consumer products companies like McDonald, Wal-Mart and other chains are entering the Eastern markets. Technology of advanced and sensitive nature like airplanes, defense as well as other components in the engineering sector is on offer by the West. There is growing demand for the technology related products. The East mostly imitates the life style of the West. The West is the moving force for the East.

Rendezvous

With the exchange of products and services, there is also exchange of human resources. The East admires the West for economic advancements as well as great achievements in the field of space and other sectors where the West is considered as a leader. With more exchange of human resources as well as tourist visits between the West and the East, the real meeting and co-production can be possible. The business of airway companies is continuing to grow with new opportunities due to this exchange process.

Products of Co-production

Setting up of new world order as well as new life style can be possible with joint efforts of the West and the East. This process of co-production will challenge many existing processes and procedures. Many products will be on offer in the market including new ways of looking at the life as well as living a happy life without stress.

Process of Co-production

This process will start creating many problems around the world. The problems of the Western world are already seen in the Eastern parts of the world including stress due to high competition, changed life styles along with change in the belief system, change in the social system and order, social problems due to changing social systems including criminal activities; the list is unending. However, the nationalists in the East are resisting the change in order to preserve the culture in the society. The conflict is continuing. The Western society will, however, start to adopt the Eastern concepts of living a peaceful life with family system. Though the techniques of mental peace and stress reduction have been accepted by the Western society, the family system is yet to evolve.

How the West Meets the East

The only way the West can successfully meets the East is through the language of love and compassion. Though the message of love and compassion is common to all religions, it is better understood among the followers of the same religion with similar cultural background or living conditions. Some times, there are conflicts arising out of the differences in customs followed by each sect or group of the same religion, and it results in hatred and bloodshed. Also, there are differences in different religions. Inter-religious dialogue is a distant dream at present. Though a lot of efforts have been made to remove the differences and focus on similarities, people with narrow personal and political interests generally get benefited by such conflicts and they keep ruling the people with 'divide and rule' policy. Universal Religion of Humanity, about which there is a lot of talk, is the only solution to this problem. Let's examine conditions in the East and the West as case studies!

CHAPTER 4

The East

Present Conditions

Typically, when we think of the East without the national boundaries but by way of the thinking process, there is a common link among the countries of the East. The East consists of many countries right from Japan, China almost up to Middle Eastern countries. The East does not include Australia, New Zealand and parts of Middle Eastern countries that do not have influence of the culture from the East. In the East, typically family ties get more importance than success in material life. The livings conditions are changing rapidly in the East with many problems faced in the West are seen in the Eastern society. The problems include stress due to high competition, changed life style, along with change in the belief system, change in the social system as well as order, social problems due to changed social system including criminal activities; the list is unending with many social implications. The social transition is continuous and challenging. Though the East refers to many countries, Indian case is discussed below being prominent among others.

Indian Conditions

Indian conditions are a reflection of average countries in the East. Though China is a leading economic power, India reflects the conditions of democratic countries. The economic and social conditions in each country are different. There are two distinct economic flows in the Indian society—old traditional workers and new workers with high income capacities such as Information Technology workers.

Old Traditional Workers

The traditional workers in the factories and businesses earn average income up to Rs.10,000 per month in advanced State of Maharashtra, and in the City of Pune (though this figure is different in each State and City). There are also workers who work with less than Rs.2,000 per month. There is huge gap in the incomes of different people. Also, the percentage of population working is less than the Western countries. The number of workers working in agriculture is reducing alarmingly with cases of suicides reported in some States due to high investment and low profit margins. The traditional workers are majority of the workforce and believe in preservation of the culture.

New Workers with High Income Capacities

Though the percentage of such workers is low at present, it is rapidly increasing creating new opportunities for businesses. 'High earn-high spend' style, however, is affecting social conditions with increasing number of 'hit and run' accident cases. Due to high spending capacity, the real estate business is booming with new state-of-art houses and apartments with Western style living conditions with new types of fixtures and furniture and swimming pools, gardens, recreation centers for occupants. The cost of such apartments in the popular area in the city of Mumbai is even higher than similar apartments in Toronto even after considering the exchange rate.

New Opportunities

There are many new opportunities for the young graduates, especially in Information Technology sector. Other sectors of the economy are also doing well with the GDP growth rate of around 8-9%. As a result of imitating the Western style of living conditions, there is a trend in the society to visit or immigrate to Western countries. Many Indians living in the West are going back to the country as it is a hub for new development and growth.

Western businesses are also taking interest in the huge emerging market of India. There are many opportunities for the West to explore in India and elsewhere in the East. India is a case in study as it is ideal case since people of different religions live in complete harmony in this democratic country. The West has many lessons to learn from this heterogeneous society with homogeneous living conditions, which is commonly known as "unity in diversity". Let's see the conditions in the West!

CHAPTER 5

The West

Present Conditions

The West typically consists of many countries from America and Europe, and Australia, New Zealand as well as the countries that do not include in the East. African countries have both East and West characteristics as they typically inherit the thoughts and social life of family ties from the East though their approach to the life is typically Western. Though economic and social conditions are different in each country, there are some similarities in terms of social conditions. The conditions in the Europe are somewhat similar to that of North America as people are following the popular culture of America in general. The Canadian case is discussed below, as it is prominent among others.

Canadian Conditions

The Canadian conditions are also reflective of American social conditions. There are two main flows of thought, and two distinct types of people *viz.* old and new immigrants. Old immigrants include French, British, Italian, Chinese, Indians and many other nationals who immigrated to Canada more than ten years ago. New immigrants are those who have come to Canada within a period of last ten years. There are two sets of different problems for both of these categories *viz.* settlement problems with cultural shock for new immigrants and second-generation problems of old immigrants. The process of settlement in Canada for new immigrants is very challenging.

New Immigrants

The new immigrants face many problems including finding a suitable job in the market as the foreign credentials are not recognized. They need to get through different processes to get Canadian experience as well as getting the right job. Canadian Governments, both Federal and Provincial, are taking steps to reduce these problems and there are many opportunities for improvements for smooth transition to Canadian conditions. One of the major problems faced by the new immigrants, especially from the East, is commonly known as 'cultural shock'. The laws in Canada are framed considering freedom and protection of privacy for every individual. Thus, the society becomes more individualistic in opposition to collective society in the East. Individualistic ways of life have their own sets of problems, especially in terms of social conditions both at schools for kids and at work for adults. The schooling system is totally different in the West compared to the East, where collective society with caring and sharing is important. The kids need to learn to live in heterogeneous society of black, brown and white. The cultural education in the East is missing in the West, and is generally done at the places of worship like temples, mosque, churches, gurudwaras and other religious centers. As a result, kids have to go through two distinct and separate schools of thought *viz.* individualistic and social living. The cases of double personality result in split or sometimes messed up mental conditions. Adults now need to learn the Western etiquette and way of living along with communication styles that is needed in the changed conditions in the West.

Old Immigrants

Though the old immigrants have successfully overcome the obstacles of settlement in Canada, their kids are generally exposed to Western way of living resulting in messed up life, if they lose the normal track of life due to break-ups between parents. Governments need to support single mothers to cope up with the rising cost of living in addition to the social support for poor people. Also, old immigrants from the East have to face separation from their families or break-ups due to changed living conditions and attitudes if the family is brought into Canada. If parents survive these problems, then they have to go through a process of transition when they have to leave their old beliefs from the East. They lose the support from the relatives who generally relieve mental stress and physical problems, commonly referred to as 'family support'. Many second generation kids leave schools before graduation or even high school education due to awareness of gap between school education and actual life conditions in Canada. Mutual ill-faith or distrust contributes to failed relationships and discontinuation of school education.

Immigrant from the West

The immigrants from the West in these both categories face the challenges in more positive manner, as the challenges in Canadian life are also a part of Western life unlike Eastern life. Of course, Europeans also face similar problems to those from the East but they have learned to live with them. Let's start the journey to Infinity by understanding the core concept of Infinity!

CHAPTER 6

Way to Infinity

What is Infinity

When we talk of Infinity, it is a state of mind where finite matters end, and there is a situation when mind loses the dual condition and one Absolute Truth prevails. Most of the saints reaching that state of mind have spoken in detail about the situation. Learned persons from any faith can explain that state of mind, as the qualities of a true religious person are the same. According to Bhagawad Geeta, one attains salvation or Moksha either by Sankhyamarg (i.e. mastering nature by understanding natural science or the Western way) or Yogamarg (i.e. mastering body and God connection or the Eastern way). (BhagwadGeeta—Ch.3-v-3/Ch.5-v-5)

State of Infinity

You may have heard the saying—"God, give me courage to change the conditions that I can; and give me patience to bear with the conditions that I can't. Most importantly, give me the wisdom to understand what I can and what I can't". In the state of Infinity, you can change the conditions that you think 'you can't change'. In this state, the wisdom and intelligence get frozen without any doubts in the mind. Faith in God leads the person through difficult conditions of life. Yogis have seen the end of 'that is' (Sat) that does not 'destroy', and 'that is not' (Asat) that does not 'live infinitely'

(BhagwadGeeta—Ch.2-v-16). Here 'Sat' is universal God, and 'Asat' is human body. All the religions believe in non-destructible existence of the universal God, and also mortal existence of human body. The duties of a knowledgeable person or a yogi are to guide ignorant people through 'leading by example' for collection and welfare of good people for good purpose. He lives selfless active life without confusing ignorant people by hypocritical methods. (BhagwadGeeta—Ch.3-v-25-26)In order to reach Infinity, it is necessary to be able to concentrate. Bhagwad Geeta calls the mental condition as 'Brahmi Sthiti' (BhagwadGeeta—Ch.2-v-72); and describes the mental conditions of the person, referred to as 'Sthitpranya' as follows (BhagwadGeeta—Ch.2-v-55-71). In order to become Sthitpranya, person has to satisfy all his sensual wishes and needs. He is happy and blissful with himself. Depression during stressful life conditions due to sorrow or expectations of happiness do not affect his mind. Love, fear and anger cannot affect him. He does not have any attachment and is not affected by love or hatred. He controls his senses from the worldly objects and remains happy with himself. When he detaches himself from the love and hatred, his soul is happy and his wisdom and intellect get frozen. He thinks in the night when others are sleeping. He becomes just like a sea when many rivers are pouring their water in the sea. As the additional water from the rivers does not affect the level of sea, the incidences in life do not affect the mental peace of such person. He does things as his duty without any expectations, self-interest and ego in a detached manner. Though it is difficult to achieve such state of Infinity in the West, it is possible to gain mental peace and happiness as a result of the process. A person without yogic qualities does not have fixed and determined way of living a life, as such, he is emotionless and as a result, he is not peaceful with himself. The problem of a confused person is that he lives in the 'past' or 'future', and ignores 'present'. This applies to men and women alike.

Why it is Difficult to Achieve Infinity

Most Western theories in natural science have outlined the nature of matter and the laws governing the matter in the nature or 'Para Prakruti', superior to 'Apara Prakruti' discussed earlier. All the objects in the nature are created either by Para or Apara Prakruti (BhagwadGeeta—Ch.7-v-5-6). The social scientists, however, have dealt with humans with the assumption that 'human being is a wanting animal'. The spiritual part starts when finite matter ends and has never been explored by natural or social scientists in the West. The great scientists like Albert Einstein have, however, realized the power of Infinity at the end of their lives. The East, on the other hand, has concentrated on the Infinity, and the medium used for such exploration was mind. Mind is very powerful and can reach anywhere at the speed higher than that of sound and light. The Rishis or spiritual scientists from the East have ignored material life being Maya or false hallucination. Due to misunderstanding the concept both in the West and in the East, it is difficult to achieve Infinity.

How to Reach Infinity

The Eastern Rishis have asked this question to those who have reached the state of Infinity. Fortunately, Indian land has produced a lot of spiritual scientists (both Munis,. unmarried, and Rushis, married) who abandoned the material life and went to the mountains or forests in search of Absolute Truth and lived in harmony with nature. The peace of mind and concentration achieved through meditation have helped them to uncover the mysteries of spiritual life. More than three thousand years ago, they have documented the process of reaching to the Absolute Truth or Infinity. The so-called mysteries of the great saints (Bible—MatthewCh.8-v-23-27) of the world like controlling the five elements of life viz. Earth (Prithvi), Water (Aap), Fire (Tej), Air (Vayu) and Space (Aakash) can be easily possible if the path of Yoga is followed to the complete discovery of knowledge.

What is Knowledge

There are two types of knowledge *viz.* Science of Nature or 'Prakruti' (Vinyan) and Science of Spirit or Soul or 'Purusha' (Nyan) (BhagwadGeeta—Ch.3-v-41). Social Science is, in fact, considered as a part of nature or 'Prakruti'. Generally speaking, unless a person fulfills his need of understanding the Natural and Social Sciences, he cannot reach to the Spiritual Science. Since Western scientists have limited themselves to the knowledge of nature they have never entered in the field of Spiritual Science. On the other hand, Eastern spiritual scientists have worked on this part of life, and ignored the Natural Sciences. Thus, when the knowledge of the West and the East is combined, it is very much possible to achieve Infinity resulting in the highest level of knowledge, peace of mind and happiness.

Which Way goes to Infinity

The only way that reaches to Infinity is through the medium of mind. The process used to make the mind powerful is meditation. The reason Yoga becoming more popular in the West is that the people are now reaching to the end of finite world, as it is full of stress and confusion. The East has referred finite world as 'Maya'. Though different cultures of the world use different ways to meditate, the East has always relied on 'yogic' way of life.

Way to Infinity

The Bhagwad Geeta in Sanskrit states, quote—

> SHREYOHI NYAN ABHYASAT, NYANAT DHYANAM
> VISHISHYATE|DHYANAT KARMA PHAL TYAGAM,
> TYAGAT SHANTI TADANANTARAM||
>
> (Ch. 12-v-12)

The meaning of this verse is that Knowledge (Nyan) is more powerful than Studies (Abhyas). Meditation (Dhyan) is superior to Knowledge (Nyan). Sacrifice (Tyag) (i.e. selfless service without expectation of gains) is superior to Meditation (Dhyan). Peace of mind (Shanti) is achieved through Sacrifice (Tyag). Quran also stresses the importance of sacrifice and devotion (Ch.108-v-2). Let's see, how to meditate using yogic methods in Swasanyoga!

CHAPTER 7

Meditation: A Way to God

Many cultures of the world prescribe different ways to meditation. It is the choice of individual to select a method of meditation. However, Yogashastra (Science of Yoga) uses following methods to set the mood for meditation (refer to Fig. 1).

Swasanyoga

'Yoga' is referred to indicate 'connecting to Supreme Power' ('yuj' verb in Sanskrit actually means 'to connect' and yoga is a noun from the verb). Yoga is practiced to reach the stage of non-duality or Unity (i.e. Oneness of matter and spirit). 'Human body' represents matter and 'mind' represents spirit (achieved through oneness of mind, wisdom, ego and conscience). Yoga is performed to get away from the duality of body, mind and wisdom leading to peace of mind. 'Swasan' means breathing. Breathing is the action of inhaling and exhaling oxygen (Prana). Swasanyoga is yogic exercise of breathing in order to reach 'yogic' state of mind.

Methods Used in Swasanyoga

There are four main methods of Swasanyoga generally used to calm down the mind through breathing. It is carried out empty stomach or four hours after drinking water or eating food and under supervision of an experienced teacher.

Yogic Concept

During inhaling (Purak), the human body (Pinda) is connected to universal God (Brahmanda); whereas while exhaling the focus comes back to the body. The process of connecting Pinda to Brahamanda is called 'Yoga'. Right nostril (Suryanadi) increases heat content in the body and left nostril (Chandranadi) reduces thought processes and emotions. Hathayoga refers to 'ha' of Suryanadi and 'tha' of Chandranadi.

(A) *PRANAKARSHAN:*

1. Deep inhaling (Purak) and exhaling (Rechak) through right nostril (Suryanadi), after closing left nostril by forefinger of right hand, and then through left nostril (Chandranadi), after closing right nostril by thumb of right hand, is called Pranakarshan (increasing oxygen in body).
2. The Purak and Rechak should be slow, deep and with constant speed.
3. The proportion of Purak and Rechak should be 1:1 increased slowly to 1:2.
4. Body posture recommended should be such that can make backbones straight and the body upright like Padmasana, Sahaj Padmasana or sitting on chair.
5. Normal breathing cycle (i.e. Purak and Rechak) is around 4 seconds or 15 times a minute depending upon the age.
6. The number of repetitions of breathing cycle should increase from 5 to 21 maximum.

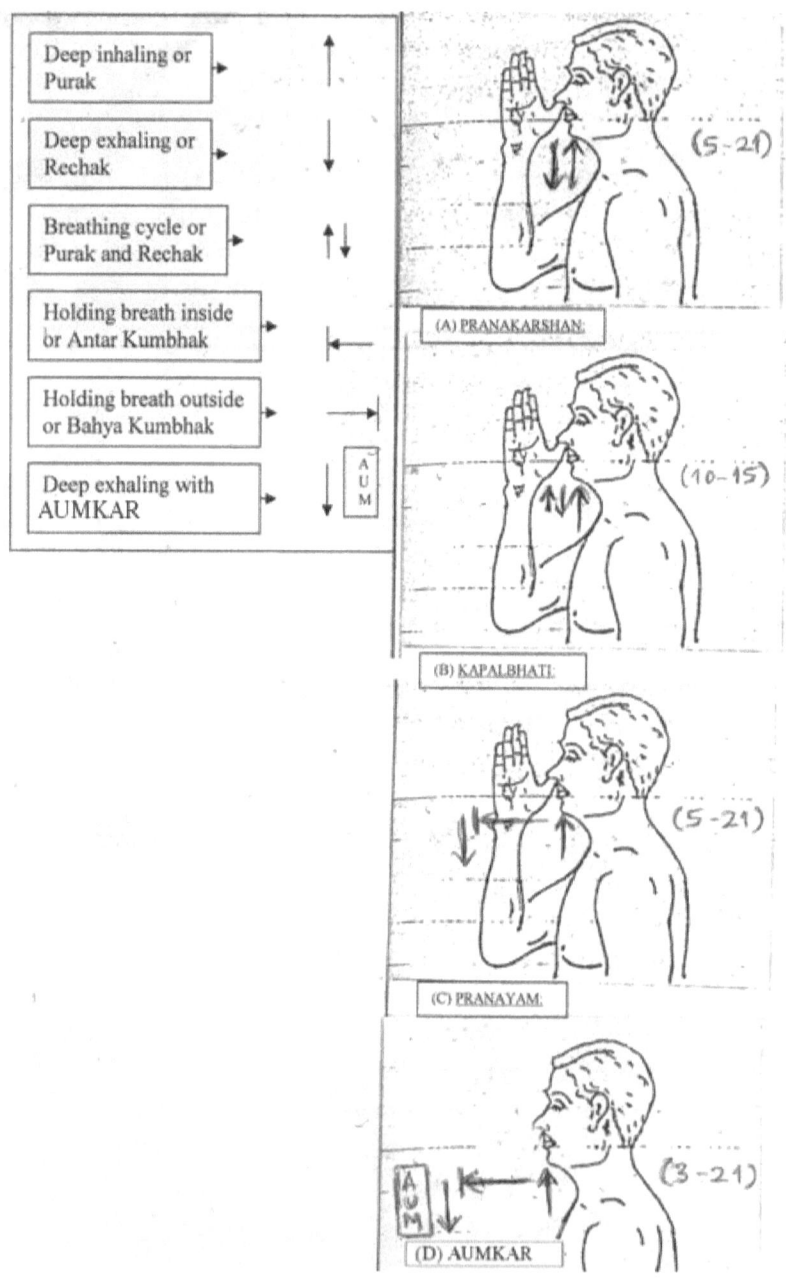

Deep inhaling or Purak	↑
Deep exhaling or Rechak	↓
Breathing cycle or Purak and Rechak	↑↓
Holding breath inside or Antar Kumbhak	⊢
Holding breath outside or Bahya Kumbhak	→
Deep exhaling with AUMKAR	↓ A U M

(A) PRANAKARSHAN: (5-21)

(B) KAPALBHATI: (10-15)

(C) PRANAYAM: (5-21)

(D) AUMKAR (3-21)

Fig.1—Methods Used in Swasanyoga

7. The time to exercise must be in the morning with an empty stomach or four hours after drinking water or eating food at other times.
8. The activation of the body through inhaling (Purak) has to be carried out from rectum to brain and deactivation through exhaling (Rechak) in reverse order.
9. The eyes should be closed and hands open on knees. The focus of mind should be on Swathisthan Chakra or pelvic area (between sexual organ and umbilicus).
10. The exercise should be carried out under supervision of an experienced teacher.

Benefits:

1. Slowing down of thought process in the mind (calming down mind).
2. Refreshing body due to excess supply of oxygen resulting in happiness, enthusiasm and energy (good for depression).
3. Purification of body germs and blood (good for weight loss and dialysis patients).
4. Longer life with health benefits especially connected to functioning of heart.

(B) *KAPALBHATI:* (Strict supervision is necessary)

1. Inhaling (Purak) deep by right nostril (Suryanadi), after closing left nostril with forefinger of right hand, followed by rapid and fast paced breathing cycle (Purak and Rechak) for about 10 to 15 repetitions is called Kapalbhati. Finally, a long and deep Purak by Suryanadi and Rechak by Chandranadi is performed. Holding breath (Kumbhak) must be done, both internally after inhaling (Purak) called 'Antar Kumbhak', and externally after exhaling (Rechak) called 'Bahya Kumbhak'. The Kumbhak should not be more than 2 to 4 seconds as per individual capacity.
2. After waiting for a minute, the same process is carried out with the left nostril (Chandranadi), after closing right nostril with thumb of right hand, with same number of repetitions. At the end, a long and deep Purak by Chandranadi and Rechak by Suryanadi is performed. Holding breath (Kumbhak) must be done, both

internally after inhaling (Purak), and externally after exhaling (Rechak). The Kumbhak should not be more than 2 to 4 seconds as per individual capacity.

3. The number of repetitions should not be increased suddenly but slowly in a step up manner. The experienced Yogi can increase the repetitions up to 108 times.
4. Kapalbhati by both nostrils simultaneously can be attempted only after eight days of daily practice with each nostril.
5. The initial Purak and Rechak should be slow, deep and with constant speed. For rapid breathing, the noise should resemble "SOHAM" i.e. HE is ME (in Sanskrit) with full concentration.
6. The proportion of Purak and Rechak should be 1:1.
7. Body posture recommended should be such that can make backbones straight and the body upright like Padmasana, Sahaj Padmasana or sitting on chair.
8. The time to exercise must be in the morning with an empty stomach or four hours after drinking water or eating food at other times.
9. The activation of the body through inhaling (Purak) must be carried out from rectum to brain and deactivation through exhaling (Rechak) in reverse order.
10. The eyes should be closed and hands open on knees. The focus of mind should be on Swathisthan Chakra or pelvic area (between sexual organ and umbilicus).
11. The exercise should be carried out under supervision of an experienced teacher.

Benefits:

1. Increased digestion capacity (good for depression, feeling not hungry or liver problems).
2. Increased efficiency of breathing (good for heart functions).
3. Purification of body germs (good for weight loss) and controlling and curing skin diseases.
4. Purification of blood (good for dialysis patients).
5. Slowing down of thought process in the mind (calming down mind).
6. Refreshing the body due to excess supply of oxygen resulting in happiness, enthusiasm and energy (good for depression).

7. Longer life with health benefits especially connected to functioning of heart, skin and liver.

(C) *PRANAYAM:*

1. The cycle of inhaling (Purak), holding the breath (Kumbhak) and exhaling (Rechak) is called Pranayam or regulating oxygen intake.
2. Inhaling (Purak) through right nostril (Suryanadi), after closing left nostril with forefinger of right hand, and after holding the breath for 8 seconds(Antar Kumbhak) as per individual capacity, while closing both nostrils with right hand thumb and forefinger, and then exhaling (Rechak) through left nostril (Chandranadi) releasing forefinger, is the first step.
3. The process is repeated by inhaling through left nostril (Chandranadi) and exhaling through right nostril (Suryanadi) after Antar Kumbhak.
4. The Purak and Rechak should be slow, deep and with constant speed.
5. The proportion of Purak and Rechak should be 1:1 increased to 1:2.
6. Body posture recommended should be such that make backnone straight and the body upright like Padmasana, Sahaj Padmasana or sitting on chair for Suryabhedan Bhasrika Pranayam.
7. Normal breathing cycle (i.e., Purak and Rechak) is around 4 seconds or 15 times a minute depending upon the age.
8. The number of repetitions of breathing cycle should increase from 5 to 21 maximum.
9. The time to exercise must be in the morning with an empty stomach or four hours after drinking water or eating food at other times.
10. The activation of the body through inhaling (Purak) must be carried out from rectum to brain and deactivation through exhaling (Rechak) in reverse order.
11. The eyes should be closed and hands open on knees. The focus of mind should be on Swathisthan Chakra or pelvic area (between sexual organ and umbilicus).
12. Pranayam in sitting condition is called 'Bhasrika Pranayam using Suryaswar' or 'Suryabhedan Bhasrika Pranayam'. 'Prathamic Ujjai

Pranayam' is carried out either in sleeping or standing condition (which is more difficult and strenuous).

13. The exercise should be carried out under supervision of an experienced teacher.

Benefits:

1. Suryabhedan Bhasrika Pranayam is useful to get rid of cough and cold (good for bronchitis patients).
2. Increased digestion capacity (good for depression, feeling not hungry or liver problems).
3. Increased breathing efficiency (good for heart functions).
4. Purifying the body of germs (good for weight loss) and controlling and curing skin diseases.
5. Purification of blood (good for dialysis patients).
6. Slowing down of thought process in the mind (calming down mind).
7. Refreshing body through excess supply of oxygen resulting in happiness, enthusiasm and energy (good for depression).
8. Longer life with health benefits especially connected to functioning of heart, skin and liver.

(D) *AUMKAR:*

1. Inhaling (Purak) deep breath and exhaling (Rechak) slowly and constantly with sound "AUM" with "A", "U" sound and "M" sound equally divided in 1:1 proportion. Here "A" stands for creation of human body (God Brahma), "U" stands for sustenance of human life (God Vishnu) and "M" stands for death of human body and unity with universal God (God Shiva). Death should be as enjoyable as life itself as is represented in the equal proportion.
2. Breathing through both nostrils (Suryanadi and Chandranadi) indicates balance of heat in body and emotions or thoughts. Suryanadi increases heat content in the body and Chandranadi reduces thought process and emotions.
3. Body posture recommended should be such that can make backbones straight and the body upright like Padmasana, Sahaj Padmasana or sitting on chair.

4. The number of repetitions of breathing cycle should increase from 3 to 21 maximum.
5. The time to exercise must be in the morning with an empty stomach or four hours after drinking water or eating food at other times.
6. The activation of the body through inhaling (Purak) has to be carried out from rectum to brain and deactivation through exhaling (Rechak) in reverse order.
7. The eyes should be closed and hands open on knees. The focus of mind should be on Swathisthan Chakra or pelvic area (between sexual organ and umbilicus).
8. The exercise should be carried out under supervision of an experienced teacher.

Benefits:

1. Increase in concentration (good for depression).
2. Slowing down of thought process in the mind (calming down mind).
3. Refreshing body due to excess supply of oxygen resulting in happiness, enthusiasm and energy (good for depression).
4. Purification of body germs and blood (good for weight loss and dialysis patients) and controlling and curing skin diseases.
5. Longer life with health benefits especially connected to functioning of heart and increased in the positive spiritual energy.

Surya Namaskar and Advanced Kriyas

After Swasanyoaga, Sun Salutation (Surya Namaskar) with certain sound is carried out. The numbers of repetitions are maximum 12 though initially one Surya Namasakar is good enough. The six Kriyas (Shadkarma) include Dhauti, Basti, Neti, Tratak, Nauli and Kapalbhati. Kapalbhati has been discussed here, but other Kriyas and Surya Namaskar are beyond the scope of this book.

Mental Yoga

The 'Mental Yoga' helps in the process of changing the mental frame for thinking. The method used for this process is meditation. The yogic tools for effective meditation have been discussed in the Swasanyoga. To change the mental frame for thinking, it is necessary to understand the connection among body, mind, wisdom and soul. The knowledge of how visible body (Pinda), including invisible mind, wisdom and soul, i.e. Kshetra (BhagwadGeeta-Ch.13-v-5-6) and person knowing complete details about the processes in the body, i.e. Kshetranya (BhagwadGeeta-Ch.13-v-1-2) or universal God are connected (yoga) is called 'Mental Yoga'. Of course, it is complicated and needs concentration to understand minute details of body processes (Pinda) and in the universe (Brahmanda) including natural processes on earth. It is achieved through connecting soul (Purusha) to universe (Para Prakruti) while breathing. The human body has both Prakruti and Purusha, and is self-contained. Soul (Purusha) is a part and parcel of God. It is believed in Hinduism that Prakruti controls both body and universe. However, since soul (God) controls Prakruti directly, in turn, God controls both body and universe by inspiring people to take actions to certain extent. Let's start journey to Infinity!

CHAPTER 8

Journey to Infinity

Bridging the Gaps of Political Activities

The political activities among different countries create opportunities as well as threats for social transition. In order to achieve full social harmony, it is necessary to increase favorable opportunities and reduce avoidable threats to mankind on the earth. The society is made up of individuals, and social change is due to the effect of individual's actions in his or her life. The journey to Infinity starts from the heart of each individual and ends in unity with God. (Bible-John Ch.15-v-3)

Four Tiers and Mixed Procreation

Hindu society had four tiers:

- Brahmin.
- Kshatriya.
- Vaishya.
- Shudra.

As per Bhagwad Geeta, the duties of four tiers or castes are based on the natural behavior or Prakruti (Ch.18-v-41). A Brahmin's natural behavior is self-satisfaction, self-control, hard working, cleanliness of mind and body, peacefulness, straight forwardness, spiritual knowledge (Nyan), wisdom based on experience and knowledge of Natural and Social Sciences (Vinyan) and faith in God. A Kshatriya's natural behavior is braveness to fight, fire like strength, courage, carefulness about safety, determination of not running away from the war like situation, donation of efforts consisting of time, labor and money and commanding the people. A Vaishya's natural behavior is engaging in agriculture, husbanding cattle including cows, and commerce of the products; whereas a Shudra's natural behavior is service to the people including health care and nursing. (BhagwadGeeta—Ch.18-v-41-44). The tiers or castes have been protected for thousands of years in Indian society. There is a specialization of genes due to marriages in same caste. As a Brahmin marrying a girl in the same caste can have child specializing in knowledge and education, the basic gene characteristics of a Brahmin. The same was true for other castes. The specialization of genes achieved through four tier system in India has been lost in Western countries. Indian society in general and Hindus, in particular have been enjoying the benefits of gene evolution and specialization. Brahmins are leading in the intelligence in academic and spiritual knowledge. Kshatriyas are leading in the intelligence in war and related techniques. Vaishyas have shown their brilliance in the intelligence in commercial knowledge and techniques. The Shudras have better qualities and the intelligence in service oriented knowledge and techniques. Over the period, the mixed procreation has resulted in combination of knowledge of these four tiers in Indian society where marriages and eggs of fertility are created among these tiers by inter-caste or inter-race marriages. However, Western society has many mixed procreations from different races. It becomes very difficult to understand the qualities of a newborn baby from the two mating partners. The basis for such understanding of qualities of a newborn baby is generally found in negative and positive spiritual energies of mating partners. If both mating partners are positive, the offspring can be positive if he comes across positive people during lifetime. However, if both mating partners are negative, then offspring generally becomes addicted to negative forces and can spread negative spiritual energy within society. The messed up offspring is the product of one negative and another positive partner. 'Satsang' or 'Company of good and positive people' is very important during the journey to Infinity.

Qualities and Characteristics of Mating Partners

The negative spiritual energy has been referred to as 'Satan', 'Demon' and 'Asur' are basically "Evil" in nature. Positive spiritual energy has been referred to as 'Allah', 'God' and 'Dev' are basically "Good" in nature. Though different religions have different terminology, the basic concepts of "Evil" and "Good" are the same. Though such qualities and characteristics have been listed at different places in both Bible and Quran, Bhagwad Geeta lists them concisely, and as such, it is referred here. The "Evil" characters show 'Tamas' qualities and "Good" characters show 'Satvic' qualities. "Human" characters show 'Rajas' qualities.

"Evil" Qualities

According to Bhagwad Geeta (Ch.14-v-8,9,13,15,18), 'Tamas' qualities beget from ignorance of spiritual knowledge. It is exhibited through indecent acts under influence of ego, laziness and sleepy attitude. It takes humans to criminal activities and non-dutiful acts due to ignorance. The person is ignorant, non-dutiful, egoistical and full of lust. The person ends up taking rebirth in animal kingdom with substandard qualities rather than as a human. As such, the person degrades himself from intelligent human being to a stupid animal.

"Evil" Characteristics

The characteristics (Ch.16-v-4-5, 7-21,23) that distinguish "Evil" are hypocritical approach or falsehood, ego, superiority complex, anger, rudeness, and ignorance of spiritual knowledge. This results in attachments to worldly objects. The person is generally confused and does not understand 'what to do' and 'what not to do' (i.e. he cannot distinguish between righteousness and sinful acts). He does not have good qualities of cleanliness, decent behavior and trustworthiness. Such people say that the world is based on lies, without any support from God, Godless and selfishness without consideration of others. They use others' efforts and enjoy worldly objects. Based on these thoughts, they end up as stupid, criminal and disrespectful people. It results in destroying the world order and people. They cannot satisfy their sexual needs, and shows qualities like hypocrisy, egoistic and carelessness, and their behavior are based on dirty thoughts and with stupid plans. To satisfy their lust, they end up doing dirty sinful jobs. They always worry for satisfying their sexual needs, and feel great need to fulfill these desires. They live with the sole objective of getting their sexual needs fulfilled. They exhibit extreme levels of expectations and anger. They use money earned by non-lawful means for fulfilling their sexual needs. They often boast like 'I have collected this much money', 'I can get even more money', 'I have defeated this enemy and can defeat others too', 'I am powerful and the happiest person', 'I am rich and belongs to family with high status in the society', 'I am the best and no one is like me', 'I will work to increase my prestige', 'I will pay to poor people', 'I will enjoy my life' and so on. Lust begets from spiritual ignorance. He lives with various stupid ideas and is interested in shameless sexual activities. They end up in Hell. They carry out social work to fulfill their egos, rudeness, satisfy false status, and show off money rather than to help people in need with a feeling of gratefulness for getting an opportunity to help others. The people with ego due to power, carelessness, sexual expectations and anger are jealous of achievements by other people; and hate God and Godly behavior by abusing them. These sinful people end up taking rebirth as demonic sinful animals. The stupid people, who are evil, never go to the Heaven but are degraded to rebirth in the animal kingdom with lower intellectual capabilities. Sex, anger and lust are doors to Hell, and need to be relinquished. The person, who behaves without control, does not get the spiritual power, happiness and cannot progress towards Moksha or Infinity.

"Evil" Symptoms

The symptoms to recognize them (Ch.17-v-4-6,10,13,18,22,28) are simple. They pray to ghost or negative spiritual energy. They are activated by falsehood, hypocrisy or ego, satisfying worldly needs, wishes, expectations, attachments, and they do not care for their own body senses and soul. They eat food that is cold, stale, stinking, left-over and non-holy. They are involved in activities not adhering to social protocol. They do not donate food, or chant the name of God. They use people for their own benefit without paying for their efforts and they do not believe in God. They behave rudely without attending to the concerns of other people with their own style of living. As a result, they not only trouble others but also themselves. They direct their efforts to destroy the lives of other people. They donate money to wrong person, at wrong time, for wrong reasons by insulting the person. Thus, the person is characterized by activities without faith in God and donating money to wrong people by insulting. Such acts are called "Asat" or evil and are not useful in material as well as spiritual advancement.

"Good" Qualities

According to Bhagwad Geeta (Ch.14-v-6,9,11,14,16-18), the 'Satvic' or "Good" qualities are self-radiating and faultless nature, and bind soul in the body by expectations of happiness and knowledge. It begets desire for happiness, and it is discernible by increasing faultless knowledge or light in the body resulting in fire like character. The person speaks out spiritual knowledge at all times. If a person dies when these qualities manifest, the person goes to Heaven that is available only to knowledgeable saints. The virtuous activities result in knowledge and "Good" or 'Satvic' character. After death, Satvic people go to Heaven. The qualities of "Good" character (Ch.16-v-1-3) are fearlessness, complete "Good" or 'Satvic' qualities, knowledge and action oriented, ready to forego money and efforts to help others, organs control, religiousness, behavior as per Dharma or righteousness, ready to take on hardships in life, straight forwardness, non-violence, truthfulness, non-anger, ready to sacrifice, peacefulness, non-enmity towards enemies, sympathy towards animals, non-lust, humbleness, shamefulness for bad activities, controlled behavior, fire like character, forgiveness, activeness, cleanliness, non-jealousy and egolessness. The 'Daivic' or "Good" qualities result in Moksha or liberation from rebirth cycle.

"Good" Characteristics

As per Bhagwad Geeta (Ch.17-v-4,5,8,11,14-17,20,23-28), 'Satvic' or "Good" people pray to God. They eat food that is full of taste, proteins, beneficial to health, body and mind. It results in increasing life span, intellectual capacities, and power. It builds strong body and mind, health, happiness and love. The sacrifice in life or 'Yagya' is carried out without any expectations but as a duty in peaceful and systematic manner, as suggested by 'Dharma' or righteousness.

"Good" Symptoms

They respect God, Brahmins or learned people, Guru or teacher and emeritus and knowledgeable people. They like cleanliness, straight forwardness, Brahmacharya or keeping away from worldly lust for sexual intercourse, and non-violence; which is referred to as 'Sharirik Tapa' or 'body purification exercise'. They speak truth but in sweet and non-hurting manner for helping others and getting results; which is referred to as 'Vachic Tapa' or 'speech purification exercise'. They keep their minds like a 'Muni' or 'Brahmachari', and control their mind by thinking of only good thoughts; which is referred to as 'Manasic Tapa' or 'mind purification exercise'. When a person without any expectation of materialistic gains follows these three Tapas or exercises with faithfulness and with yogic wisdom it's called 'Satvic Tapa' or 'Good exercise'. They donate time, money, labor and other efforts as if it is their duty, and offer them to other persons who have not helped them but considering rightness or justifiability of place, time and personality in terms of reason that creates need for help as well as personality traits considered 'good' by society; it's called 'Satvic Dan' or 'donation for good cause'.

Aum, Tat and Sat

The Aum, Tat and Sat are three ways to refer to Brahma or Prajapati or the God of Human Creation. He has created 'Brahmins' or 'knowledgeable people', 'Vedas' or 'knowledge' and 'Yagya' or 'sacrifice'. As world started with utterance of 'Aum', the people praying Brahma start 'Yagya' or 'sacrifice', 'Dan' or 'donation', 'Tapa' or 'hard work' in life by uttering 'Aum'. People expecting Moksha or liberation from rebirth cycle work without expectations of gains and carry out 'Yagya', 'Tapa' and 'Dan' by uttering 'Tat'. Reality and goodness refer to by using word 'Sat'. Also, auspicious work is called as 'Sat'. The state of doing 'Yagya', 'Tapa' and 'Dan' and also the related action is called 'Sat'. Actions without faith in God like 'Yagya' or 'sacrifice', 'Dan' or 'donation' and 'Tapa' or 'hard work' is called 'Asat'. These are neither useful in the materialistic life nor eternal life.

Yagya, Tapa and Dan

As per Bhagwad Geeta (Ch.18-v-5,6,9,20,23,26,30,33,36,37), the actions of 'Yagya' or 'sacrifice', 'Dan' or 'donation' and 'Tapa' or 'hard work' are necessary for all wise and knowledgeable person as it results in cleanliness of conscious mind and removal of dirt from the mind. These actions need to be carried out without any expectations of gains or attachment to the actions resulting in ego or status. When these actions are carried out in a detached manner and without any expectation of gains, the 'sacrifice' is called 'Satvic Tyag' or 'sacrifice for good cause'.

Nyan, Karma and Karta

The knowledge with which different animals and human beings carry out life with similar, non-decaying and non-exclusive nature of behaviour, the knowledge is called 'Satvic Nyan' or 'Good knowledge'. When actions are performed without expectations in detached manner without love or hate, it is called 'Satvic Karma' or 'Good action'. When the person is detached, without ego, courageous and enthusiastic and does not get affected by success or failure, he is called 'Satvic Karta' or 'Good doer'.

Buddhi, Dhruti and Sukh

The wisdom and intellect that understands well which thing is 'needed to be done' or 'not needed to be done', and for righteousness, which action is 'right' and which is 'wrong', for which things one 'needs' to be faithful or which 'need not', which thing can result in 'attachment' and which lead to 'detachment' or Moksha (i.e. liberation from rebirth cycles); it is called 'Satvic Buddhi' or 'Good wisdom'. The firm belief due to yogic state drives the actions of mind, soul and senses. The drive power of a person due to firm belief in God in yogic state of performing actions of mind, soul and senses is called 'Satvic Dhruti' or 'Good cause drive' (i.e. 'Good Spirit'). The happiness after repeated experience results in feeling nice, and results in the end of the sorrows in life, and though it feels like poison when started, finally results in Amrit or nectar of immortality, as a result of blissful condition of mind, intellect and soul is called 'Satvic Sukh' or 'Good happiness'. The Rajas or Human qualities are placed in these two extremes of "Evil" and "Good"; which basically represent human desire for ego, status and praise by others.

Way to Achieve Mental Peace through Procreation

Though mental peace is difficult to achieve in the stressful Western life, meditation and procreation of mating partners with positive spiritual energies can make a major difference in the Western countries. It is difficult, however, to understand the positive energy of a partner. In a society where people are busy meeting their basic needs, it is very difficult to think of specialized projects such as procreation. Also, it is difficult to define person with positive spiritual energy objectively. Mostly, babies are procreated when the two partners are in tender age when it is not possible to identify positive energy traits in a person. Sometimes the relationships are the result of economic compulsions, when it is not possible to control the characteristics of an offspring. Most of the problems of Western world are due to uncontrolled procreation and helpless upbringing of a child in stressful life conditions. Though such conditions are not as stressful as in the Western world, in the East, the stress is seen in industrialized countries like Japan, China, Hong Kong, or even India to some extent. The effect of stress in many situations is less compared to the West due to spiritual practices in the East.

Spiritual Basis for Same Sex Marriages

The two parts of a human being *viz.* Prakruti (Female) and Purusha (Male) are also characterized by tenderness of a female and strength of a male. In fact, one can even see in a female, male characteristics of strength, or female characteristics of tenderness in a male. Same sex marriages can find a base in these qualities if one of the partners has qualities of opposite sex.

Advances in the West

Most of the advances made in the West are in Natural and Social Sciences or Prakruti. Traditionally, the Easterns have regarded Prakruti as Maya or false hallucinations. Also, it was easy to work with Purusha with the help of Yogamarg rather then Prakruti using Sankyamarg, which was difficult (BhagwadGeeta—Ch.12-v-5). Some experts have worked on Prakruti consisting of five elements:

- Earth(Prithvi),
- Water(Aap),

- Fire(Tej),
- Air(Vayu)
- Space(Akash)
- And mind, wisdom and ego (BhagwadGeeta—Ch.7-v-4).

Rushis or spiritual scientists have done a great job on materialistic developments in the East a few thousand years ago. Western societies have made great achievements in controlling nature using Natural and Social Science or Vinyan. The advances in the West have created techniques to control first five elements (Earth, Water, Fire, Air and Space) of Prakruti to some extent, but they could never be able to control the last three *viz.* mind, wisdom and ego that are controlled by Purusha. The problems of the West are due to the last three.

Advances in the East

Most of the spiritual leaders focused on Purusha or soul. The medium used for studies of soul has been mind. The experts like Patanjali, who brought the principles of Yoga (Patanjali Sutra) into existence, have developed methods for mind control through meditation. Patanjali studied different animals and used their postures for the benefit of human health, both physical and mental. He defined the physical postures of Yoga based on the name of the animal e.g. Matsyasan (fish), Marjarasan (cat), Sinhamudra (lion's face) and so on, some times objects e.g. Halasan (plough), Dhanurasan (bow), Naukasan (boat) or even the part of the body used for the posture e.g. Sarvangasan (whole body), Shirshasan (head). There are eight components (Ashtang) of Yoga, however, three main pre-requisite for Yoga as medication are

- Niyama (rules or principles of life),
- Sadhana (Yoga, Kriyas and Mental Yoga)
- Ahar (eating habits).

Easterners have even discovered that the first five elements of Prukruti (Earth, Water, Fire, Air and Space) have been transformed and sensed by human body through what is known as 'Tanmantras'. Earth (Prithvi) is sensed through smell (Gandha). Water (Aap) is sensed through taste (Rasa). Fire (Teja) is sensed through sight (Rupa). Air (Vayu) is sensed through touch (Sparsha) and Space (Akash) is sensed through sound (Shabda). These Tanmantras are very useful in relationship building and lovemaking. Speech or communication (i.e. sound) is very important during this process. A lot of research has gone in to such theories, but unfortunately, it was locked up in the literature written in Sanskrit and forgotten over the time. The present times characterized by stressful life conditions need studies and development of these advancements in Spiritual Science of the East.

Reaching Infinity or Moksha

As believed by the East, the only way to peace and happiness is through development of Spiritual Science. The debates of whether Prakruti or Science of Nature (Vinyan) is more important than Purusha or Science of Spirit (Nyan) are worthless as the two (i.e. Natural and Spiritual Sciences) are complementary to each other and cannot exist without the existence of other. It is just like for the continuation of life on earth and reproduction process of human being, both male (Purusha) and female (Prakruti) are necessary. The Natural Sciences exist only while there is life on the earth. Only after reaching to the end of Natural Sciences, can one enter Spiritual Science. To reach the lifeless stage in the Spiritual Science, it is necessary to understand both these sciences (BhagwadGeeta-Ch.6-v-8) when the mind can reach to a stage of fulfilled wishes. The ultimate aim of human existence is to unite with God so that the cycle of rebirth can be ended.

Path to Reach Infinity

Bhagwad Geeta in Sanskrit states—

TAPASWIBHYODHIKO YOGI, NYANIBHYO API MATO ADHIKAHA|KARMIBHYA CHA ADHIKO YOGI, TASMAT YOGI BHAV ARJUN|| (Ch.6-v-46)

Yogi is more valuable than Tapaswi (hard working spiritual saint). Yogi is more valuable than Nyani (knowledgeable saint). Yogi is also more valuable than Karmic (spiritual person with expectations). That is why, be a Yogi, oh Arjun!

North America needs more Yogis, who can deliver and not just speak, in order to reach Infinity rather than Yoga teachers or instructors, though they are also necessary.

3-0

INDEX

COMING ATTRACTION

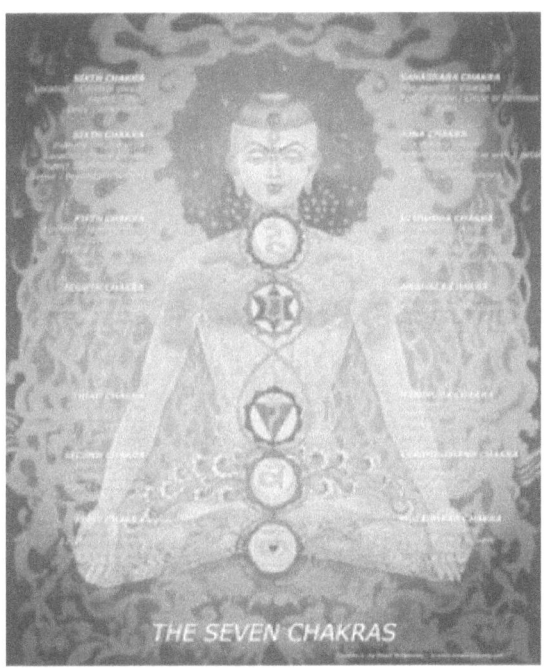

source: http://www.sanatansociety.org/yoga_and_meditation/
seven_chakras.htm

Journey within Seven Chakras

By Aadeshnath

During yogic Journey to Infinity, it is necessary to understand the effects of Mental and Physical Yoga. This book is first attempt to help understand actual stage in self-realization. Kundalini Yoga made simple and brief for yoga and meditational practioners.

www.ingramcontent.com/pod-product-compliance
Lightning Source LLC
Chambersburg PA
CBHW021252280526
45784CB00005B/2336